Fine Tuning
The Human
Machine

by

Harold Elrick, M.D., F.A.C.P.

D1367513

San Diego, California
February 1993
First Edition

Fine Tuning The Human Machine

How to achieve an optimal lifestyle

Printed in the United States of America
by
ICAN Press
616 Third Avenue
Chula Vista, CA 91910

Contributing ICAN Staff

James Zadeh . . . . Publisher
Dahk Knox . . . . Editor-in-Chief
Josette Rice . . . . .Senior Editor
Dave Carroll . . . . Overseas Marketing Director
Mary Mahoney . . . . Editor
Robert Hernandez . . . . . .Editorial Assistant
Jan Knox . . . . Writer
Ben Guico . . . . Layout
Carlos Toth . . . . Illustrator
Ernest Veil . . . . Press Manager
Isela Martinez . . . . Production Manager
Patricia Medina . . . . Production Assistant
Ray Bermudez . . . . .Production Assistant
Lonnie Lewis . . . . Administrative Assistant
Patricia Godsoe . . . . Administrative Assistant
Lou Nestler . . . . .Video Productions Manager
Lester Knox . . . . Video Productions Assistant

Printed in the United States of America
Library of Congress
Library of Congress Cataloging-in-Publication data
ISBN # 1-881116-17-04

Copyright February © 1993
by Harold Elrick, M.D., F.A.C.P.

> The study of the human body and its requirements for optimal health should be made a basic principle in all educational effort . . . each individual should regard his health as sacredly as his character.
>
> **Frederick Rossiter, M. D.**

> Every man is not only the architect of his own character, but is the builder and custodian of his own health and physical well being.

Acknowledgments

Special acknowledgment is due to Dr. Dahk Knox, Josette Rice, other ICAN Press staff members, and Carlos Toth for his illustrations and cover.

Special appreciation is due Mary H. Mahoney for her excellent editing contributions and advice on the original manuscript, and to Patricia Godsoe for her desktop publishing efforts.

TABLE OF CONTENTS

Foreword

This is one of the best promotional ideas I've encountered. What could be more logical than a do-it-yourself users maintenance manual for yourself?

Dr. Elrick has been a long-time practitioner of health promotion for himself and his patients. I had the privilege a few years ago to review with him the benefits his patients had gained by following his prescription for healthy living. I was enormously impressed with what he had accomplished. Improvements in patients with the chronic diseases of aging, by following Dr. Elrick's logical program of self care, resulted in reduced high blood pressure, improvements in coronary heart disease, arthritis, diabetes control, obesity and other such ailments. Patients were able to avoid medications or be controlled with smaller doses. His results were better than those obtained in large national clinical trials with drugs.

Health costs have risen through the ceiling in part because physicians wait in their offices or hospitals until patients seek help for their manifest illnesses. The medical profession then responds with ingenious, high-cost technological interventions which all too often palliate rather than cure the illnesses. If physicians were to make a serious effort to prevent these illnesses, the health of the public would be better served and probably at lesser cost.

We physicians have unfortunately contributed to the mistaken current belief that one can indulge in whatever lifestyle he or she wishes and then, when illness strikes, medicine will make available a pill or operation to erase the adverse health effects of a lifetime of self-abuse. We need to disabuse the public of this fantasy. The route to improved personal and public health is not through the pharmacy and the operating theatre but via the sage advice provided in this little maintenance manual.

Help yourself to personal health and well-being!

Alexander Leaf, M.D.

Jackson Professor of Clinical
Medicine, Emeritus
Harvard Medical School

and

Distinguished Physician
Veterans Affairs
Boston, Massachusetts

**Health is nature's reward for getting
into harmony with her laws.
It is the law of life
to maintain one's health
or suffer the consequences.**

A. A. Montapert

Preface

When you purchase an automobile, computer, camera, washing machine or any other machine, it comes with an owner's manual for maintaining proper functioning. The human being is faced with a challenging paradox. We are the most complex of all creations, with the greatest potential for abundant life, and yet we have no owner's manual. All individuals must discover how best to care for themselves with occasional assistance from a variety of "experts." We seek the advice of professionals only after a parts failure or breakdown occurs.

This book is to be used as an instructional manual for the operation and maintenance of the human "machine." You'll get the best results and longest service from your body by taking the advice of this book and incorporating it into your daily life.

Using the analogy of the automobile, the topics are: fuel, maintenance, avoidance of road hazards, and tune-ups.

The ideas expressed herein are based on the studies of 10 population groups. They are characterized by exceptional longevity, freedom from the major diseases, and/or superior health-fitness. Countries represented in this study were: U.S.A., Ecuador, Russia, Hunsa, Japan, China, Bali, and Mexico.

Introduction

Each of us has been given the priceless gift of life and a one-of-a-kind mind and body with unlimited potential. The physical durability of the human being has been proven by the fact that more than 30,000 Americans are over 100 years old. The stamina of the human being has been demonstrated by the Tarahumara Indians of Mexico, who are able to run 200 or more miles continuously. A human brain's capability is over 1,000 times that of the most sophisticated computers. The human capacity for learning, compassion, loving, creativity, artistic or scientific achievement, moral behavior, joy, and selfless deeds, is without bounds. These abilities of the human being far exceed that of any other animal species. And yet the vast majority of individuals achieve only a minute fraction of this vast potential.

The average life span of Americans is only 75 years. Many individuals are partially or totally disabled physically or mentally many years before their deaths. Coincident with this premature deterioration is often a deterioration of financial status and standard of living; e. g., a large majority of retirees are financially dependent on others. The discrepancy between the potential and the actual is indeed striking. It is especially deplorable because this premature rate of deterioration is commonly believed and widely accepted as **normal** aging.

Fortunately, some of the major causes of this situation are known and correctable, such as, acceptance of "normal" goals and standards, ignorance of the mind/body potential, and negative attitudes.

The principal goal of this manual is to describe how you can come much closer to achieving your potential through optimal care of your mind and body and by avoidance of destructive factors. The table on Page 5 shows the important differences between *normal* and *optimal* standards and goals.

Why should optimal health be everyone's top priority?

The best answer to this question was given more than 2,000 years ago by a Greek physician named Herophilus. He said:

"When Health is absent,
Wisdom cannot reveal itself,
Art cannot become manifest,
Strength cannot fight,
Wealth becomes useless, and
Intelligence cannot be applied."

Aim for the optimal not the normal.

"The best six doctors anywhere
and no one can deny it,
are Sunshine, Water, Rest and Air,
Exercise and Diet.
These six doctors will attend
if only you are willing;
your ills they'll mend,
your cares they'll attend,
and charge you not a shilling."

Unknown Author

Decide what you want, decide
what you are willing to
to exchange for it.
Establish your priorities and
go to work.
H. L. Hunt

The Normal/Optimal Concept

The normal/optimal characteristics of health illustrated in this chart show marked differences between normal (average) and optimal (best achievable) goals.

Normal standards were derived from the general American public, which has a high incidence of major diseases: cardiovascular diseases, hypertension, obesity, diabetes, etc. They represent the C grade or average (mediocre) level of health-fitness. In contrast, the optimal standards were derived from population groups with the highest level of health-fitness and, thus, represent the A grade or highest level of health-fitness.

The "normal" individual has a mediocre level of health and performance and a high risk for the major, fatal diseases. "Optimal " health means the highest achievable level of health and performance with the lowest risk for serious diseases.

> **It is possible for every man to achieve betterment of the quality of his life.**

1993 Standards: Normal vs. Optimal

(According to Elrick)

	NORMAL	OPTIMAL
Diet - Daily Restrictions/ Requirements	Xs: Cal, Fat, Prot, Chol, Sodium	Cal: 1500 to 2400 Fat: less than 20 gm Protein: 40-80 gm Chol: less than 150 mg
	Deficiency: Fiber, Calcium	Calcium: 1.5 gm Sodium: less than 2 gm Fiber: 30-50 gm
Exercise	None to Occasional	Daily: 1 hour Minimum
Rest	Sleep: 6-8 hours	Sleep: 8-9 hours + Nap: 30-60 min. daily
Bowel movements/day	0-2	2-4
Smoking	Common	Abstinence
Alcohol & Other Drugs	Very Common	Abstinence
Heart Rate/ minute	70-90/minute (untrained)	Less than 50/minute (trained)
Blood Pressure	140/90 or less	120/80 or less
Percentage Body Fat	Female: 20-30 % Male: 15-25 %	Female: 10-19 % Male: 5-14 %
Cholesterol (mg%)	150 - 250	125 - 175
HDL Chol (mg%)	Greater than 35	Greater than 40
Triglycerides (mg%)	Less than 150	Less than 100
O_2 MAX - ml/kg/minute	Less than 30 (untrained)	Greater than 40 (trained)

5

Optimal Weight Table

Currently used Height-Weight tables have several shortcomings that render them inaccurate and misleading. They were derived from the general American public which is notorious for its prevalence of overnutrition, obesity, sedentary life, frequent drug and medication usage and high incidence of diseases associated with unhealthy living habits (Life Style diseases). Part of the data was obtained by questionnaire, i.e. the subjects submitted their heights and weights obtained in an uncontrolled manner. The division into 3 types of frame is arbitrary and the ranges at each height are very broad. Finally, the wide differences in lean body mass (muscle and bone) are not taken into account.

From the standpoint of health-fitness, the fat mass (% body fat) is the most important parameter rather than the total body weight. The following table is based on acceptable models of optimal health-fitness, namely, competitive and recreational endurance athletes (primarily distance runners aged 15-80) of both sexes, vigorous active individuals from 7 countries of all ages who had no evidence of major life style diseases, and female beauty contest winners from all over the world. The table does not apply to individuals with extremes of muscle or bone mass.

Optimal Weight Table
(according to Elrick)

Height (in)	Weight (lb)			
	Women		Men	
	OH[1]	OH+OP[2]	OH[1]	OH+OP[2]
60	90-98	88-96	95-105	92-102
61	94-102	91-99	100-110	96-106
62	98-106	94-102	105-115	100-110
63	102-110	96-104	110-120	105-115
64	106-114	100-108	115-125	110-120
65	110-118	102-110	120-130	115-125
66	113-120	105-115	125-135	120-130
67	116-125	110-120	130-140	125-135
68	120-130	115-125	135-145	130-140
69	125-135	120-130	140-150	130-145
70	130-140	125-135	145-155	135-150
71	135-145	130-140	150-160	140-155
72	140-150	135-145	155-165	145-160

1 Optimal Health (and Appearance): Women (15-19% fat) Men (10-15% fat).
2 Optimal Health + Optimal Performance: Women (less than 15% fat) Men (less than 10% fat).

Performance

The graph below relates physical performance to the chronological age of a human being. It illustrates the difference between normal (average) individuals and those who are optimal in health (at various ages). Note that optimally healthy individuals have a higher level of performance at all ages and live longer. The performance level of Olympic champions is shown for comparison.

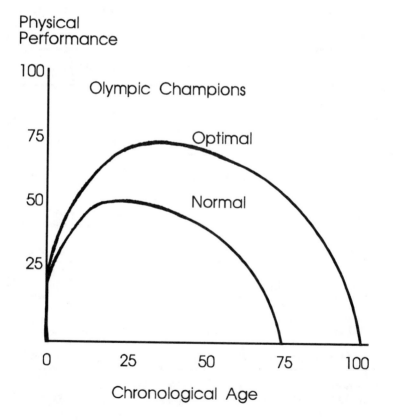

Aging

Chronological age is a risk factor for many diseases. However, large differences (variability) in the rate of aging and functional capacity at any age make it an unreliable factor. The great variability in the rate of aging, primarily due to differences in living habits, often results in considerable differences between chronological and functional (physiological) ages. Thus, we see 40 year olds who perform like 60 year olds and 60 year olds who perform like 40 year olds. Clearly, functional capacity or age is of equal (or more) importance to health and longevity as chronological age. Thus, functional age estimation or evaluation is an important part of health-fitness evaluation and for predicting individual active life span. This is in addition to the other factors, such as heredity, sex, blood chemistry, blood pressure, body fat, and living patterns.

Aging in the "normal" American follows a typical pattern in the absence of intervention of health promoting techniques. Maximal health-fitness occurs early (age 12-16) and declines progressively with age. By the age of 60, partial disability has developed and often progressed to total disability by the age of 70 with death occurring in the mid-seventies in a nursing home or in the home of relatives. Individuals who are able to continue a productive career and maintain their living standards independently at the age of 80 or more are a rarity in our society. In contrast, there is considerable epidemiological evidence that the maintenance of an independent, active and productive life and career to the age of about 100 is possible and not a rarity. Such individuals have a different life style than the typical inhabitant of the U.S. and other industrial nations.

The search for the "Fountain of Youth" in one form or another is universal. Nearly everyone desires and dreams of remaining "young" until death. Actually this is not an impossible dream if the fixation on chronological age is discarded and the concept of functional age is accepted. Many individuals (including many well-known people) have lived a full, active working life until they died (suddenly) at ages greater than 90.

In order to estimate functional age, certain indicators must be evaluated, namely, posture, body movement and appearance (skin, hair and expression) in addition to the parameters of the health-fitness profile described on page 5.

Characteristics of Youthfulness:

- Optimal living habits, fitness level (physical performance) and blood chemistry
- Trim body (optimal body fat) and firm muscles
- Vigorous, flexible, agile body movements
- Skin: smooth, thick, healthy color, minimal wrinkles
- Facial expression: alert, receptive, relaxed, attentive
- Minimal (or no) graying of hair.

The conventional (normal) methods of achieving youthfulness are superficial and artificial. It may be called the health spa approach. It is basically a "crash course program": hair styling and coloring, facial cream and other "beauty aids", clothes, fast weight loss diets and exercise programs, cosmetic surgery of face, breasts and removal of excess fat.

Remarkable results with respect to acquiring the characteristics of youthful appearance can be achieved by a program of optimal living habits combined with posture-gait-movement conditioning. Youthful facial expression is achieved by developing the optimal attitudes and beliefs (pages 46-49).

Estimating how "young" you are is based on chronological, functional, risk factor and appearance ages. The relative importance of each of these aspects of age is difficult to determine. Accordingly, we arbitrarily consider them of equal value and derive final age from an average of the four ages. For example, an individual with a chronological age of 70, a functional age of 40, a risk factor age of 35 and an appearance age of 60 is 51 years young. [70+40+35+60=205/4=51]. Furthermore, if the individual has the optimal health-fitness profile, he or she has a PAY (predicted active years) of 30 years (70-100) of life remaining.

CONCEPT OF AGING &
LONGEVITY 1993
According to Elrick

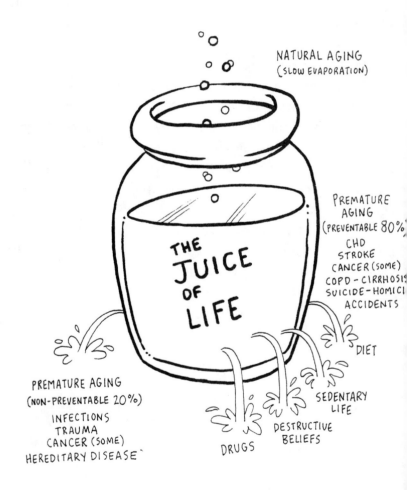

Fuel (Food)

General Principles

Before purchasing food products, read the ingredients on the label. If you do not know what the ingredients are, look them up in a nutrition reference book. In particular, note the calorie, fat, and sodium content of each serving and the serving size.

Learn to convert grams (gm) into calories: 1 gram of fat = 9 calories, 1 gram of alcohol = 7 calories, 1 gram of carbohydrate or protein = 4 calories.

Avoid high-fat and high-sodium foods, such as butter, margarine, nuts, fried foods, egg yolks, pastries, candy, cookies, seeds, regular dairy products, mayonnaise, peanut butter, most salad dressings, and many canned foods.

Eat frequently (6 or more times a day) in small quantities: "nibbling or grazing."

Eat slowly, chewing thoroughly, putting the eating utensil down until each mouthful is swallowed. Spend at least 20 minutes eating a meal and 5-10 minutes per snack.

When eating at a restaurant: (a) Order only grilled, baked, or broiled foods; (b) Avoid sauces, gravies, salad dressings, and soups; (c) Eat only half or less of the meal. Take the remainder home to eat at a later time.

Keep a food diary until optimal goals are achieved.

Specifics

Eat small amounts (100-400 calories) every 2 1/2 to 3 hours between 7:00 a.m. and 10:00 p.m.

Daily foods should include

(a)   Fruit: 3-5 servings per day (fresh or frozen).

(b)   Vegetables: 4-6 servings per day (fresh, frozen, or canned). Canned vegetables should be washed for two minutes with tap water to remove sodium.

(c)   Pasta, rice, beans, cereals, and breads (nonfat, low-sodium, sugarfree): 6-10 servings per day

(d)   Nonfat dairy products (milk, yogurt, cheese): 2-5 servings per day.

The number of servings for each of the preceding foods depends on the percentage of body fat and weight. If these measurements are above the optimal (page 5), the lowest number of servings is recommended until optimal body fat is achieved. Thereafter, increase servings to numbers that maintain optimal body fat and weight.

Restrict the various animal products (meat, fish, and poultry) to 7 oz. or less per week.

Restrict certain foods to small servings once a month or less. These include: pizza, hot dogs, peanut butter, hamburgers, nuts, seeds, and fried foods.

Restrict the total daily intake of any type of fat to less than 20 grams by consuming foods that contain 2 grams or less fat per serving.

Restrict desserts to 100 calories or less.

Eat cereals and breads that contain no fat or sugar and less than 150 mg. of sodium per serving.

Restrict total daily intake of sodium to less than 2 grams.

Use the many tasty substitutes for the most common high-calorie foods: nonfat salad dressings, egg substitutes, salt substitutes, nonfat pastries, nonfat frozen desserts, nonalcoholic wine and beer, and carob powder (for chocolate).

Avoid the use of vitamin, mineral, or protein supplements.

If tempted to eat an unhealthy food, resist the impulse for two minutes: such cravings usually last less than two minutes.

Your daily caloric intake should range between 1,200 and 2,500, depending on your percent of body fat and physical activity.

Drink a glass of water every time food is eaten.

Use spices generously to add flavor (without calories) to meals, particularly garlic, pepper, mustard, onion, oregano, dill, thyme, lemon juice, cumin, basil, cilantro, curry, and hot peppers.

Do not keep unhealthy foods in the house.

	AMERICAN DIET	**OPTIMAL DIET**
Calories	2500-3500	1000-2500
Protein	100-140 gm	40-75 gm
Fat	100-140 gm	10-20 gm
Carbohydrate	300-400 gm	150-450 gm
Cholesterol	600-1000 gm	0-150 gm
Sodium (salt)	5-10 gm (10-20 gm)	1-2 gm (2-4 gm)
Calcium	300-600 mg	800-1500 mg
Fiber	less than 15 gm	25-40 gm

The seven essentials of health are:
Fresh air, good food, pure water, sunshine,
exercise, abundant rest, and power of the mind!
Nature is God's physician.

Maintenance of Body and Mind

The Body

"Those who think they have no time for physical exercise will sooner or later have to find time for illness."
                                        The Earl of Darby, 1873

The human body thrives on movement and deteriorates with inactivity. Exercise stimulates blood flow and tissue growth in muscle and bone. Inactivity results in tissue atrophy and a reduced functioning of muscle, bone, and brain. Physical movement gives pleasure and stimulates creativity. It also relieves the fatigue of nervous tension and sedentary activity. Thus, the importance of maximum body movement cannot be overemphasized.

The achievement of this goal requires the intermittent, moderate use of all muscle groups throughout the day:

- Brisk walking for daily activities (chores, shopping, errands, visiting, recreation).

- Restrict sitting activities to eating, learning, writing, and essential driving.

- Frequent use of isometric exercises for all muscle groups while engaged in sitting activities: using upper body, abdominal, and leg muscles.

- Hourly body movement for 5-10 minutes while engaged in prolonged sitting activities.

- An exercise program characterized by a variety of three or more activities, that are pleasurable and suitable for life long use.

- Emphasis on endurance activities (vigorous walking, running, cycling, swimming): five days per week for a minimum of one hour (four percent of the day). Nonendurance, activities such as racquet or team sports, rowing, or skiing are options on the remaining days. The objective is to do at least one or two activities every day.

- An exercise period to relieve any fatigue resulting from sedentary work or nervous tension.

- Stretching and relaxing exercises for a few minutes at least once daily (pages 21-36).

- Posture and back exercises daily (pages 37-42).

Additional Measures:

Care of teeth and gums: Brush, floss, or use a toothpick after eating. Schedule dental check-ups two to three times a year.

Care of skin: Protect yourself from the sun by wearing proper clothing and hats. Use sunblock cream.

Care of feet: Wear proper shaped shoes and use proper foot alignment. Change shoes and socks frequently. Dry between your toes. Cut nails straight across. Remove calluses with pumice, **not** razor blades. Go barefoot indoors. Use open sandals as much as possible outdoors.

Adequate rest: Get 8-9 hours sleep every night from 10:00-10:30 p.m. to 6:00-6:30 a.m., plus 30-60 minutes of rest every afternoon.

Learn to measure your heart rate at your wrist, neck, and groin. Record your heart rate at rest, at work, and during and following your exercise session. Objectives: to get the lowest possible rate at rest (40-50/min.); to get 120-150/min. during exercise and decrease to 100/min. two minutes after exercise.

Test your cardiovascular, pulmonary, musculo, and skeletal fitness periodically by means of the 12-minute test (page 43).

The objective of the optimal exercise prescription is to achieve the individual's maximal potential of physical fitness. This level varies very widely from person to person but is predictable with considerable accuracy by an analysis of the health-fitness evaluation and by the response to conditioning. It depends on the age, genetic endowment, motivation, perseverance, and previous physical conditioning at work, recreation and sports.

The criteria of the optimal program regardless of the cited factors can be summarized by the acronym: **DF ALIVE**

D means **daily**: to establish the habit of exercise

F means **fun:** a necessity for compliance

A means **availability**: close to home or work place

L means **life long**: easily done the entire life (eliminates team activities)

I means **independently**: not dependent on other people or facilities

V means **variety**: of physical activities (walking, running, swimming, cycling, etc.)

E means **endurance**: most important program aspect.

In summary, the objective is to establish a life long habit of enjoyable physical exertion that leads to maximal individual fitness.

Stretching Exercises

It is important to perform proper stretching exercises before any increased physical activity. The purpose of stretching before a hard workout is to prevent straining the muscles.

The stretching exercises shown on the next few pages are the "top of the line," because after a few sessions, you'll experience increased flexibility, strength, and circulation. You will also experience less fatigue if you perform these stretching exercises after a hard workout such as walking, jogging or swimming.

> **Your body is a temple of the Holy Spirit**
> **who is in you, whom you have from God,**
> **and that you are not your own . . .**
> **therefore, glorify God in your body.**
>
> **The Holy Bible (1 Corinthians 6:19)**

Ballet Stretch

Stand about three feet away from a wall or support. Your feet must be shoulder width apart and in alignment with your hips. Place your left foot forward to the point where you'll feel a pull on your leg muscles in the back of your right leg while keeping your heel down. Extend your right arm, placing your right hand on the wall. Your right foot should be in alignment with your hand, extended as far back as you can, while keeping your heel flat. Now, starting with your waist, twist your body to the left, with your left hand touching your waist. Look to the left. Hold that position for at least one minute. Repeat that movement, reversing your leg and hand positions. This exercise stretches the muscles of your arms, legs, and back. Repeat this exercise six times.

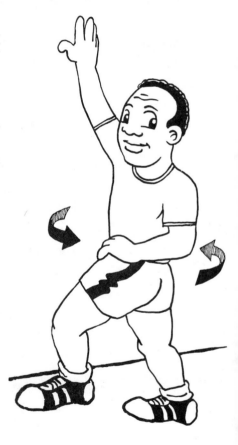

Hip Extender Stretch

Sit on the floor. Put the soles of your feet together. Keep your back straight. Place your hands on each of your ankles, with your elbows pressing against your knees. Apply gentle pressure downward and hold for three seconds. Release your ankles. Repeat this exercise twelve times.

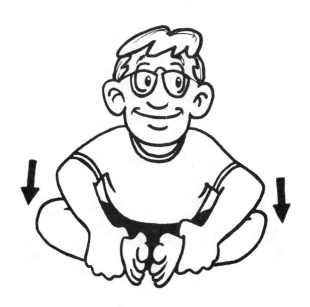

Hip   Flexor

Sit on the floor and put the soles of your feet together. Keep your back straight. Place your hands on each of your ankles with your elbows pressing against your knees. Try to bring your knees together while resisting with your arms and elbows. Hold this position for three seconds. Release your ankles and repeat this exercise 12 times. Now repeat the hip extender stretch and alternate with three sets of hip flexors.

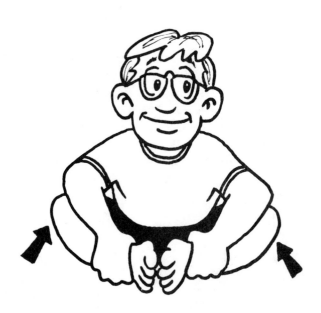

Hamstring Stretch - Right Leg

Lie on your back on the floor. Keep your left leg straight. Raise your right leg, bending your knee. Now try to straighten your right leg at the knee. Hold your right foot flat and parallel with the ceiling. Flex your ankle. Hold this position for three seconds. Release and lower your leg from its bent position at the knee. Repeat this exercise 12 times. Do two sets.

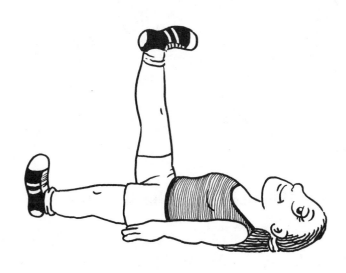

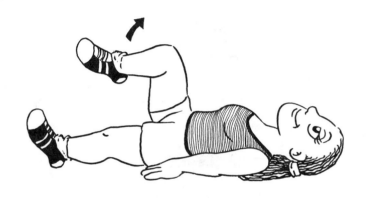

Hamstring Stretch - Left Leg

Lie on your back on the floor. Keep your right leg straight.
Raise your left leg, bending your knee. Now try to straighten
your left leg at the knee. Hold your left foot flat and parallel
with the ceiling. Flex your ankle. Hold this position for
three seconds. Release and lower your leg from its bent position
at the knee. Repeat this exercise 12 times. Do two sets.

Relaxation Exercises

Directions: All of these exercises should be done very slowly and in a relaxed manner. They can be done on any firm surface, such as a carpeted floor or bed. They should be executed in a slow motion. Hold each position for approximately three seconds before doing the next movement.

Head Rolls

Lie on your back with your knees bent. Rotate your head slowly from side to side. Repeat this exercise 12 times for each side.

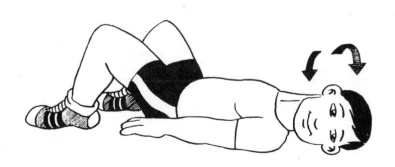

Shoulder/Head Roll

Repeat your head roll, but move your shoulder downward. As you turn your head to the right, move your right shoulder downward. Do the same with your left shoulder as you rotate your head to the left. Repeat this exercise 12 times for each side.

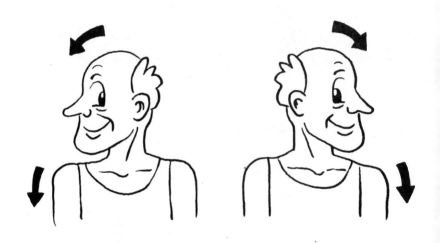

Knee Flex

Lie on your back with knees bent. Slowly bring the right knee toward your chest and clasp the knee with both hands. Next, bring the left knee toward the chest and clasp with both hands. Release the right knee and place the right foot on the floor. Then release the left knee and place the left foot on the floor. Repeat this exercise 12 times on each side.

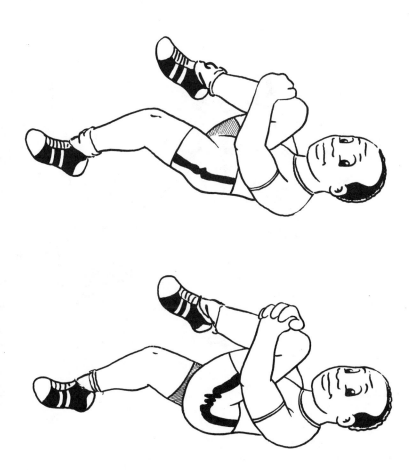

Knee/Hip   Rotation

Lie on your back with both of your knees bent. Bring your knees towards your chest and clasp a knee with each hand. Now, move the knees in a circle to the right 12 times. Then move the knees to the left 12 times.

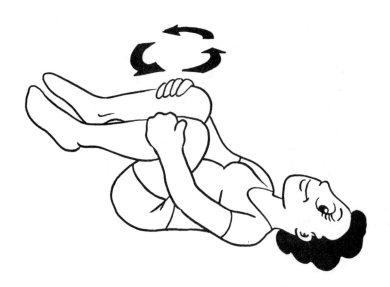

Opposite Elbow To Knee

Lie on your back with your knees bent. In one continuous motion, bring the right knee and the left elbow together. Then do the same movement on the opposite side. Repeat this exercise 12 times on each side.

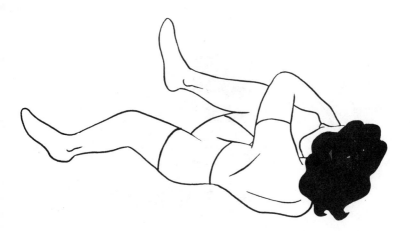

Bridge

Lie on your back with your knees bent. Lift your buttocks and shoulders off the floor. This will extend your spine. Repeat this exercise six times.

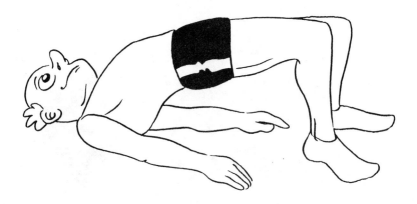

Leg Slide

Lie on your right side. Bring your left leg in toward your chest. Then slide your leg along the floor, back behind the your body. Repeat this exercise 12 times. Now lie on your left side. Move your right leg 12 times, doing this same exercise.

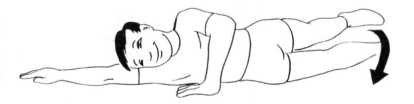

Cat/Dog

Get on your hands and knees. Arch your back like a cat. Your neck should be relaxed with your head down. Your back should be rounded. Repeat this position 12 times.

To go into the dog position, reverse the curvature of your back. The head should move upwards. Repeat this position 12 times.

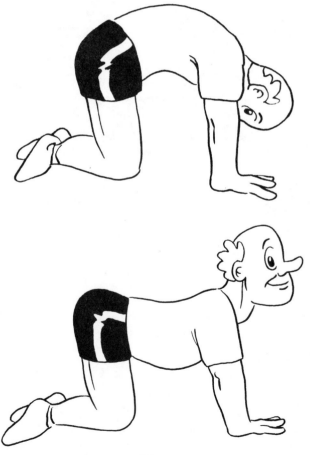

Crawling

Crawl on your hands and knees for approximately 12 seconds.

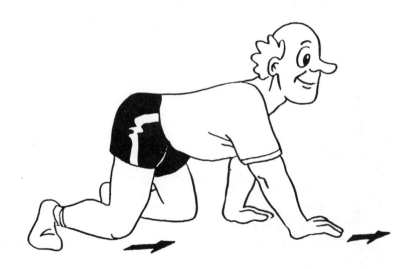

Chair Bend

Sit straight upwards in a chair or on a couch. Bend over with your hands moving from your thighs downwards to the front of your toes. Now reverse your hand movement. Go backwards, up your legs, until you return to your original sitting position. Repeat this exercise 12 times.

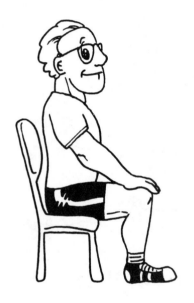

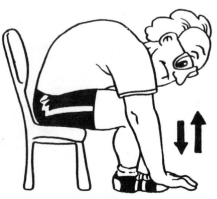

Posture And Back Exercises

Standing Pelvic Tilt

Stand with your heels two to three inches away from a wall. The entire backside of your body, including your shoulders and head, should be touching the wall. Tighten your stomach muscles and flatten the small of your back against the wall. Your pelvis should tilt backwards. Hold this position for three seconds. Repeat this exercise 12 times.

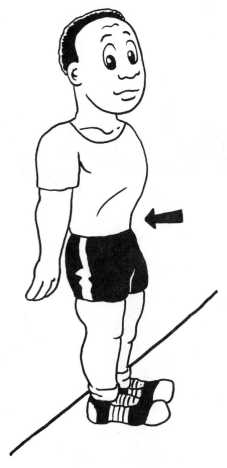

Supine Pelvic Tilt

Lie with your back completely touching the floor. Tighten your stomach muscles and flatten the small of your back. Hold this position for three seconds. Repeat this exercise 12 times.

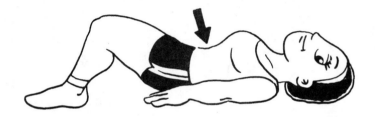

Rocking Horse

Lie with your back on the floor. Clasp your knees with your hands. Gently raise your shoulders and head toward your knees. Now gently rock back and forth for two minutes.

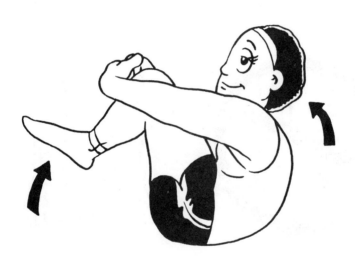

Leg Alignment

During daily activities, such as sitting, walking, and running, continuously keep your feet straight and parallel. Think of a car's proper front wheel alignment. Keep your back straight.

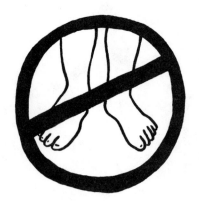 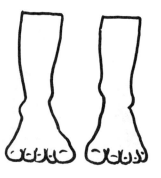

Deep Breath

Periodically during the day, take deep breaths and your body will automatically straighten. Your posture will automatically correct itself. As you release air, maintain that correct posture. The advantage of this technique is to achieve erect posture anytime, anywhere. As the day progresses and you feel like you're slumping, take another deep breath.

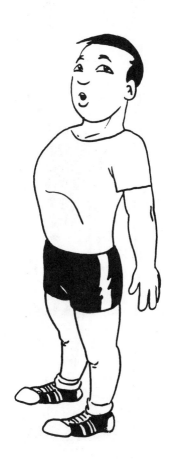

Imaging

Whenever possible, remember how straight you stand while getting your height measured and you will automatically stand straight and tall.

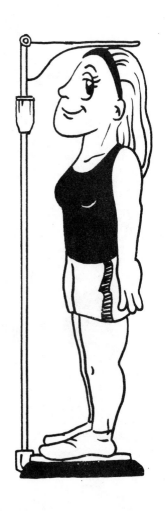

Health-Fitness Measurement
Twelve-Minute Test

This test is simple to perform and requires no special equipment or assistance. It is best done on a standard quarter-mile track, such as the type of tracks found at high schools and colleges. If no running tracks are available, a suitable distance can be measured on a level country road or field, using a car or bicycle odometer. It may also be performed indoors on a measured track or floor. Running or gym clothes should be used.

Because the test is for maximum physical capacity, the subject should make a maximum effort to cover as much distance as possible during a twelve minute period. He or she may, of course, stop, walk, jog, or run, depending on the level of fitness and ability.

> **The image you see of yourself,**
> **when your eyes are closed,**
> **is most likely the image**
> **you display to the world.**
> **If you want to be what you see**
> **inside your mind,**
> **you must first realize and visualize**
> **that possibility**
> **becoming a true reality.**
> **Dahk Knox**

Classification of Cardio-

(Adapted from Cooper

Grade

I. Very poor: Patients with cardiovascular-pulmonary diseases, marked obesity, and musculoskeletal diseases.

II. Poor: No disease, but markedly impaired cardiovascular-pulmonary fitness or obesity.

III. Borderline: The "weekend" athlete.

IV. Fair: Those engaged in nonendurance sports on a fairly regular basis and the ex-athlete.

V. Good: The level reached by many after 6-12 months of a good endurance exercise program. The recommended goal for most people.

VI. Very Good: The level achieved by a minority of people after a year or more of a good endurance exercise program. Recommended level for the competitive athlete (nonendurance sports.)

VII. Superlative: The competition endurance athlete.

Vascular-Pulmonary Fitness

12-minute test)

Distance (miles) covered in 12 minutes	Maximal O_2 consumption ml/kg/min
< 0.5	< 24
0.5 - 1.0	24 - 28
1.0 - 1.24	28.1 - 34
1.25 -1.49	34.1 - 42
1.50 - 1.74	42.1 - 52
1.75 - 2.0	52.1 - 60
> 2.0	> 60

The Mind

Our attitudes, beliefs, and thoughts govern our lives and are expressed by our feelings and behavior. They are shaped by our experiences from early childhood. Nonetheless, each of us has 100% control of our thoughts. Therefore, it follows that we can reshape our attitudes just as we can reshape our bodies. The following attitudes are characteristic of very successful people in a wide variety of human endeavors. They serve as models to emulate.

Optimism

Feel good about yourself, your work, your relationships, and the world in general. Expect the best to happen. Find the good in every event or situation.

Excellence

Do your very best in every task you undertake. Always "put your best foot forward."

Control and Responsibility

Be in control of your life and take full responsibility for everything that happens. Accept both credit and blame.

Goals

Establish goals for today, tomorrow, and the coming months and years ahead. Put those goals in clear, specific written form.

Be flexible enough to make changes along the way to reaching those goals. Perseverance is the key to goal achievement. It requires understanding that failures along the way are indispensable, because they teach us how to succeed.

Work

Spend the time and effort required to discover the type of work you love to do, and devote your working life to this endeavor.

Respect

Feel, show, and express respect for yourself, other people, animals, the environment, the law, morals, and especially ideas and customs that differ from your own.

Reactions

Realize and accept that the most important aspect of every event in your life is your own reaction to it, rather than the event itself.

Time Organization

Realize that time is the limiting factor in life. Organize time well to allow you to spend it on your highest priorities.

Self-Esteem

The way you feel about yourself -your reputation with yourself- determines how well you'll do in every aspect of your life. That reputation is enhanced by an awareness of your unlimited potential as a unique human being. This reputation is reinforced by repeated successes and personal growth in a goal-oriented life. Increasing your self-esteem is a continuous, highly desirable process that leads to continuing achievement and satisfaction.

Human Relationships

Getting along well with all kinds of people is a source of great joy, rewards, and successes in life. Everyone's business is "people" business. Treating people the way they want to be treated is the basis for establishing and maintaining valuable personal and professional relationships. The ability to forgive others as well as yourself is essential for enduring loving relationships and avoiding destructive, negative emotions.

> **In the province of the mind,**
> **what one believes to be true either**
> **is true or becomes true.**
>
> **John Lilly**

Life-style Rating Sheet

	Initial	1 mo.	2 mo.	3 mo.	6 mo.	12 mo.	18 mo.
Adherence to diet (%)							
Adherence to exercise (%)							
Attitude change (%)							
Elimination of drugs (%)							
Weight							
Blood Pressure							
Resting Pulse							
1 mile walk test							
12 minute test							
Bowel movements							
Rest (8 hours)							
(Siesta)							
Fit feeling							
Energy							
Self-esteem							
Well being							
Teaching ability							
Other changes noted							
Blood							
Cholesterol							
HDL Cholesterol							
Triglycerides							
Glucose							
Uric Acid							
Urine							
Sodium							
Specific Gravity							

49

Since the mind is a specific biocomputer,
it needs specific instructions and directions.
The reason most people never reach
their goals is that they don't define them,
learn about them, or ever seriously consider
them as believable or achievable.
Winners can tell you where they are going,
what they plan to do along the way, and who
will be sharing the adventure with them.

Dennis Waitley

Hazards Along the Road

The major hazards or obstacles on the road to achievement, happiness, and "fulfillment of potential in life" fall into the following categories:

Destructive Attitudes (Negative Emotions)

Over 50 obstacles that thwart success have been identified. The principal ones are: pessimism, worry, fear, doubt, anger, hostility, hate, revenge, distrust, resentment, and suspicion. They usually result from focusing on the consequences of failure or assuming responsibility for the actions of others.

Mythical Barriers

Age, race, religion, skin color, physical size or appearance, heredity, environment, lack of education, financial or social status, childhood abuse, and physical handicaps need not be obstacles to a highly successful, productive, rewarding life. On the contrary, they have often acted as powerful motivations for outstanding achievements and happiness.

Vocabulary "Garbage"

The human mind has many characteristics of a computer with limitless capabilities. Thus, it's important to control what is put into it. The computer rule GIGO (garbage in garbage out), applies to the mind. Such words as " I can't," "I have to," "I'm no good at" or any other expressions of self-depreciation (or a lack of self-control) must not be entered into your "mind computer" by way of thoughts or oral expressions. Once negative thoughts are entered, they become your reality whether actually true or not.

Activities That Harm Relationships

Arguing or quibbling
Criticism of self and others
Offering unsolicited advice
Attempting to change others
Inability to forgive self and others

Drug Usage

Drugs may be divided into several categories:

*   Medical (prescription)
*   OTC (over-the-counter)
*   Alcohol and tobacco
*   Coffee and tea
*   Soda drinks containing caffeine or phosphoric acid
*   Illegal drugs
*   Supplements (vitamins, minerals, proteins, hormones)

All of these substances, except for the supplements, are foreign to the human body and therefore they are potential poisons that occasionally have beneficial side effects. The supplements are also potential poisons because they are usually used in doses that far exceed normal requirements.

The only justifications for risking the potentially damaging or fatal side effects of these substances are:

(1)   They are proven to be life-saving or life-prolonging in the situation in which they are being used.

(2)   They improve the quality of life in a terminal illness.

(3)   They relieve severe, intolerable pain that is temporary in nature, e.g., during or after surgery.

(4)   They restore a proven deficiency of a natural, vital substance (hormomes or vitamin) and are used in physiological doses.

> **In reality, moral rules are directions for running the human machine. Every moral rule is there to prevent a breakdown, or a strain, or a friction, in running that machine.**
>
> **C. S. Lewis**

Living Habits & Disease

Faulty Habits	Diseases
1. **Wrong Diet**	Obesity
	Hypertension
	Atherosclerosis
	Lipid Disorders
2. **Sedentary Life**	Diabetes
	Cancer
3. **Smoking**	Cancer
	Cardiovascular Diseases
	Emphysema
	Accidents
	Cirrhosis
	Cancer
4. **Drugs (Alcohol, etc.)**	Heart Disease
	Brain Disease
5. **Destructive Beliefs**	Suicide
	Homicide
	Mental Diseases

THE LIFESTYLE DISEASES

Elrick's Iceberg: Unseen perils that can cause our shipwreck

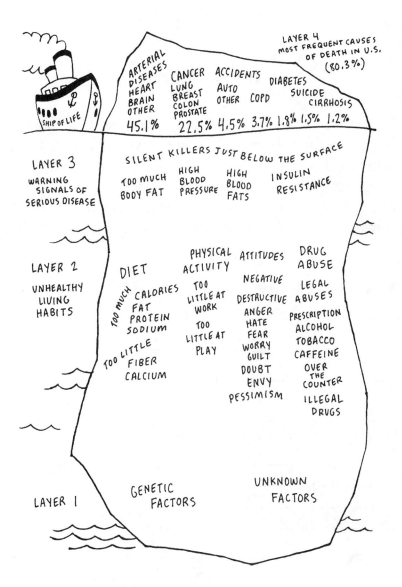

SHIP OF LIFE

LAYER 4
MOST FREQUENT CAUSES
OF DEATH IN U.S.
(80.3%)

ARTERIAL DISEASES HEART BRAIN OTHER	CANCER LUNG BREAST COLON PROSTATE	ACCIDENTS AUTO OTHER	COPD	DIABETES	SUICIDE	CIRRHOSIS
45.1%	22.5%	4.5%	3.7%	1.8%	1.5%	1.2%

LAYER 3

WARNING SIGNALS OF SERIOUS DISEASE

SILENT KILLERS JUST BELOW THE SURFACE

TOO MUCH BODY FAT   HIGH BLOOD PRESSURE   HIGH BLOOD FATS   INSULIN RESISTANCE

LAYER 2

UNHEALTHY LIVING HABITS

DIET
TOO MUCH CALORIES FAT PROTEIN SODIUM
TOO LITTLE FIBER CALCIUM

PHYSICAL ACTIVITY
TOO LITTLE AT WORK
TOO LITTLE AT PLAY

ATTITUDES
NEGATIVE DESTRUCTIVE ANGER HATE FEAR WORRY GUILT DOUBT ENVY PESSIMISM

DRUG ABUSE
LEGAL ABUSES
PRESCRIPTION ALCOHOL TOBACCO CAFFEINE OVER THE COUNTER
ILLEGAL DRUGS

LAYER 1

GENETIC FACTORS

UNKNOWN FACTORS

55

Personal Commitment
to Change

Introduction

To become committed to a better life, you must make a personal decision to change certain behaviors that inhibit you from reaching and achieving your fullest potential. Below are several statements that require your honest input. Consider your answers before you respond to each statement. Be ready to make a personal commitment for change.

An attitude or behavior I wish to change:

_____

_____

_____

_____

Benefits to me by making this change:

_____

_____

_____

_____

Three things I must do to make the change:

_____

_____

_____

The date by which I will accomplish the change:

_____

Three steps I will take this week:

_____

_____

_____

Three things that will ensure my success:

_____

_____

_____

It's a funny thing about life; if you refuse to accept anything but the best, you very often get it.

Somerset Mangham

How to Reshape Attitudes and Habits

(1) Your desired change must be precisely characterized, written down, and read daily.

(2) You must have a very strong desire to change your behavior, acquire a positive attitude, or generate new habits.

(3) You must make a firm commitment to change, without second thoughts or reservations.

(4) You must have a strong conviction that you can do it, never doubting your will to succeed.

(5) Your new attitude must be mentally practiced and rehearsed: your outward behavior should be repeated daily until your change becomes established.

We become what we think about.
You can determine what you think about,
therefore, you can determine what you become.

Earl Nightingale & Napoleon Hill

Tune-Up (Check-Ups)

Periodic check-ups of your body functions are necessary for detecting malfunctioning too subtle to be perceived by you. Indeed, serious illness may be present in an early stage at a time when the individual feels and functions well. Feeling well in itself is not reliable evidence of good health. There are countless examples recorded in the daily newspapers of people who have suffered a catastrophic illness with no warning, e.g., heart attack, stroke, appearance of a malignant tumor, or sudden death.

Tests detecting early evidence of serious disease, in time for effective measures to prevent or control a disastrous outcome, are actually few in number, relatively simple, and inexpensive. They are:

* Blood pressure, heart rate, weight, and waist measurement

* Body fat percentage

* Blood chemistry:
  SMA 24,
  HDL cholesterol

* Complete blood counts

* Urine analysis

* Pap smear for all women over 20 years old

* Mammograms for all women over 45 years old

* Posture and gait analysis

* Cardiovascular fitness measurement: 12-minute test (pages 43-45).

The standards and goals for optimal health-fitness are shown on page 5. If you achieve these standards, you'll ensure substantial decrease of risk for serious disability, disease, and premature death.

Summary

In Short : The Optimal Life Style

The optimal life style is designed to enable the majority of individuals to achieve their innate full potential of a productive, joy-filled, satisfying, disease-free, healthy life. Such a life was symbolized in Oliver Wendell Holmes' famous poem, **The Deacon's Masterpiece: The Wonderful One Hoss Shay.** This poem is a tale of a vehicle constructed of the finest materials available. It gave excellent service without parts failure for 100 years, then suddenly and unexpectedly fell apart.

(1)   **Eating Pattern** (pages 13-16)

       Content: Fruits, vegetables, cereals, grains, pasta, and nonfat dairy products daily.
Meat, fish, and poultry (3-4 oz. servings) two times weekly or one ounce per day.
Fat: 20 gm or less/day.
Sodium: 1-2 gm/day
Calcium: 1-1.5 gm/day
Amount: 1000-1200 calories/day if body fat is greater than optimal. 1500-2500 calories/day if body fat is optimal.
Schedule: 6 or more feedings/day of 100-400 calories each at two- to three-hour intervals.

(2)   **Body Movement/Exercise** (pages 17-42)

Daily and throughout the day.
Minimal sitting and standing.
Variety: endurance, strength, stretching, and relaxing.
two or more types daily.

(3)   **Optimal attitudes** (pages 46-49).

(4)   **Avoidance of all drugs** (page 52).

(4)   **Achievement of the Optimal Health-Fitness Standards** (page 5).

> **Most of our ills come from our wrong acts and wrong thinking, and such a life-style inhibits our potential growth, prosperity and well being.**

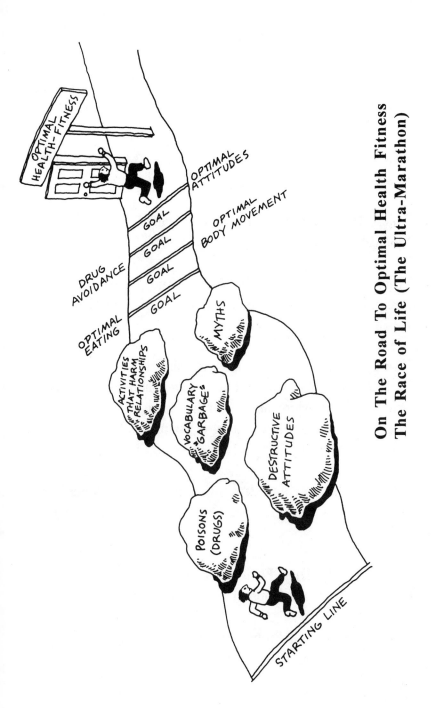

**On The Road To Optimal Health Fitness
The Race of Life (The Ultra-Marathon)**

References

Elrick, H.: **Living Longer and Better.** (Guide to Optimal Health) Mountain View, CA, World Publications, 1978.

Elrick, H.:"A New Definition of Health," Journal National Medical Association <u>72</u>: 695-699 1980

Elrick, H.: **How to Eat for Health and Pleasure.** (Optimal Recipes and Menus) Bonita, CA, Foundation for Optimal Health and Longevity, 1980.

Elrick, H.: "Life Style Diseases: Results of Non-Drug Therapy in 120 cases, Physical Activity, Aging and Sports," Vol. 1. Scientific and Medical Research. Harris, R. & Harris, S. Education Center for the Study of Aging. Albany, New York, NY, 1989.

Elrick, H.:**Therapy and Prevention of Disease without Drugs.** Bonita, CA, Foundation for Optimal Health and Longevity, 1990.

Elrick, H.: **The Dual Focus Method of Patient Care.** Bonita, CA Foundation for Optimal Health and Longevity, 1991.

Elrick, H.: "Health Promotion for Diseases of Industrialized Nations," Medicine, Exercise, Nutrition and Health. May-June 1992.

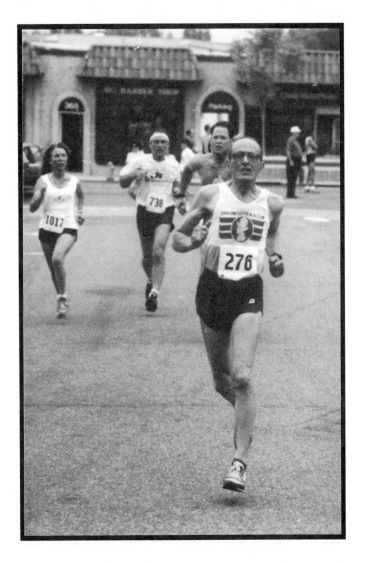

Dr. Harold Elrick began his running career and commitment to achievable optimal health in 1968. Since then, he has competed in hundreds of races, from 1 mile to 26 mile marathons, and won many age group awards. The above picture of Dr. Elrick (#276) was taken during a 10 kilometer (6.2 mile) race when he was 72 years old.